GASTROENTERITIS

LEARNING THE KNOWN TREATMENTS FOR

BELLY FLU

DR. DAWN RAY

Contents

CHAPTER ONE

INTRODUCTION

Gastroenteritis is an contamination resulting from the infection and contamination of the digestive device. Normal signs and symptoms and signs encompass abdominal cramps, diarrhoea and vomiting. In masses of cases, the situation heals itself within a few days.

The principle trouble of gastroenteritis is dehydration, but this will be avoided if the fluid misplaced in vomit and diarrhoea is replaced. Someone stricken by excessive gastroenteritis may additionally additionally want fluids administered intravenously (without delay into the bloodstream via a vein – the setup is regularly known as a 'drip'). Some of the causes of gastroenteritis embody viruses, bacteria, bacterial pollutants, parasites, unique chemical substances and some drugs.

When you have diarrhea and vomiting, you could say you have the "belly flu." these signs and symptoms and symptoms frequently are due to a situation called gastroenteritis.

With gastroenteritis, your stomach and intestines are angry and inflamed. The cause is usually a viral or bacterial infection.

Viral gastroenteritis is an intestinal infection that includes symptoms and signs and symptoms including watery diarrhea, belly cramps, nausea or vomiting, and on occasion fever.

The most common manner to develop viral gastroenteritis — regularly called belly flu — is through contact with an inflamed man or woman or thru ingesting infected food or water. If you're otherwise healthful, you will probably get higher with out headaches. However for toddlers, older adults and those with compromised immune systems, viral gastroenteritis may be lethal.

There's no effective remedy for viral gastroenteritis, so prevention is prime. Avoid meals and water that may be contaminated and wash your fingers very well and often.

Belly flu, viral gastroenteritis, is a viral infection in your digestive machine. It causes gastrointestinal signs like vomiting and diarrhea. It's typically quick, but may be very contagious.

Belly flu is a viral infection that affects your belly and intestines. The scientific term is viral gastroenteritis. "Gastro" way belly and "input" method small gut. "Itis" method contamination, this is typically because of an infection. And "viral" manner that a virulent disease has caused the infection.

Belly flu causes gastrointestinal (GI) symptoms like diarrhea, belly cramps and nausea. You could also call it a "stomach computer virus." A stomach worm isn't usually an endemic — once in a while it's micro organism or a parasite — but anyhow, the signs and symptoms are comparable. You may no longer have the capability to inform if your pc virus is a virulent disease or not.

Signs of gastroenteritis

The signs and symptoms of gastroenteritis can embody:

Lack of urge for food

Bloating

Nausea

Vomiting

Belly cramps

Belly ache

Diarrhoea

Bloody stools (poo) – in a few cases

Pus in the stools – in a few times

Typically feeling sick – which include lethargy and body aches.

Reasons of gastroenteritis

There are numerous matters that would reason gastroenteritis, together with:

Viruses – which includes norovirus, calicivirus, rotavirus, astrovirus and adenovirus

Bacteria – including the Campylobacter bacterium

Parasites – which encompass Entamoeba histolytica, Giardia lamblia and Cryptosporidium

Bacterial toxins – the micro organism

themselves don't motive illness, however their toxic via-products can contaminate meals. A few traces of staphylococcal bacteria produce pollution which could reason gastroenteritis

Chemical materials – lead poisoning, for instance, can cause gastroenteritis

Medication – certain medicinal drug (at the side of antibiotics), can cause gastroenteritis in inclined human beings.

When to look a medical doctor

In case you're an person, name your health care enterprise if:

You are not able to maintain liquids down for twenty-4 hours

You've been vomiting or having diarrhea for additonal than days

You're vomiting blood

You are dehydrated — signs and symptoms and symptoms of dehydration consist of excessive thirst, dry mouth, deep yellow urine or little or no urine, and intense weak spot, dizziness or lightheadedness

You phrase blood in your bowel actions

You've got severe stomach ache

You have a fever above 104 F (40 C)

For infants and youngsters

See your infant's health care company right away in case your infant:

Has a fever of 102 F (38.Nine C) or better

Appears worn-out or very irritable

Is in a variety of ache or ache

Has bloody diarrhea

Appears dehydrated — look ahead to signs and symptoms of dehydration in sick infants and kids through evaluating how loads they drink and urinate with how lots is ordinary for them, and watching for signs and signs in conjunction with a dry mouth, thirst and crying with out tears

If you have an little one, take into account that even as spitting up can be an regular incidence in your child, vomiting isn't. Toddlers vomit for an expansion of motives, many of which may additionally require scientific interest.

Name your child's medical doctor right away in case your little one:

Has vomiting that is not unusual

Hasn't had a moist diaper in six hours

Has bloody stools or severe diarrhea

Has a sunken gentle spot (fontanel) at the top of his or her head

Has a dry mouth or cries with out tears

Is unusually sleepy, drowsy or unresponsive

What does the begin of belly flu sense like?

For many people, belly flu symptoms seem to return on all of sudden and out of nowhere. You can throw up or have diarrhea usually on that first day. Symptoms and signs stand up one to two days once you had been exposed to the virus. Happily, they're usually over just as speedy, resolving in a single to two days.

What are the ranges of belly flu?

The degrees of belly flu infection are:

Publicity. You're most in all likelihood to get the belly flu from someone in your network, specifically in a closed environment like a faculty, nursing domestic or cruise ship. Thinking about signs make the effort to growth, you'll probable pay interest about a virulent disease later, while you were exposed.

Incubation. When you've shriveled the virus, it'll begin replicating interior your frame. This is the incubation period. You gained't have signs and symptoms till the virus replicates sufficient to alert your immune gadget. This normally takes some days, counting on the virus.

Acute contamination. Viral gastroenteritis is an acute contamination, which means that it's unexpected and transient. Whilst your immune tool registers the hazard, it turns on an inflammatory response to clean the virus. That is what reasons signs and symptoms and signs of illness. While it succeeds, the signs and symptoms will save you.

Recovery. You'll note your signs lessening while your immune gadget has gained the battle against the virus. In the end, your signs will forestall, and also you'll experience better. However you could hold to shed the virus to your poop (stool) for some days, because of this which you're despite the fact that contagious.

How prolonged does stomach flu remaining?

Belly flu commonly simplest lasts a few days, however it is able to last up to each week or in extreme cases. People with weaker immune structures can also have a harder time defeating the virus, and it is able to take longer.

Is stomach flu contagious?

Positive, it's very contagious. You should limit your contact with others when you have it. If you live with others, ensure to clean your palms regularly and disinfect shared surfaces, specifically within the bathroom.

How long is the stomach flu contagious?

You're maximum contagious sooner or later of the extreme segment of the contamination (when you have symptoms and symptoms) and for some days after. But, you may nevertheless be a touch contagious for up to two weeks once you have better.

Infectious gastroenteritis

Infectious gastroenteritis is as a result of viruses, bacteria or parasites. In each case, infection takes place even as the agent is ingested, usually by way of eating or eating. A number of the not unusual varieties of infectious gastroenteritis encompass:

Escherichia coli contamination – that could be a common trouble for visitors to international places with terrible sanitation. Infection is because of ingesting infected water or ingesting contaminated raw stop end result and greens.

Campylobacter infection – the bacteria are found in animal faeces (poo) and raw meat, mainly chook. Contamination is due to, for instance, eating inflamed meals or water, eating undercooked meat (especially bird), and now not washing your hands after handling infected animals.

Cryptosporidium infection – parasites are placed in the bowels of people and animals. Contamination is because of, as an example, swimming in a infected pool and by means of risk swallowing water, or through touch with infected animals. An inflamed man or woman may additionally moreover spread the parasites to food or surfaces in the occasion that they don't wash their hands after going to the bathroom.

Giardiasis – parasite infection of the bowel. Contamination is due to, as an example, eating inflamed water, handling inflamed animals or converting the nappy of an infected infant and no longer washing your fingers afterwards.

Salmonellosis – bacteria are decided in animal faeces. Contamination is as a result of consuming contaminated food or managing inflamed animals.

CHAPTER TWO

An inflamed man or woman may moreover spread the bacteria to one of a kind human beings or surfaces thru now not washing their arms well.

Shigellosis – bacteria are placed in human faeces. An inflamed character can also spread the bacteria to food or surfaces in the event that they don't wash their palms after going to the rest room.

Viral gastroenteritis – contamination is resulting from individual-to-character touch collectively with touching inflamed hands, faeces or vomit, or through using ingesting infected water or food.

Analysis of gastroenteritis

It's miles important to set up the motive, as exclusive forms of gastroenteritis respond to important treatments. Diagnostic strategies may moreover encompass:

Clinical records

Physical exam

Blood assessments

Stool assessments.

Treatment for gastroenteritis

Remedy relies upon at the reason, however may additionally include:

Plenty of fluids.

Oral rehydration beverages, available out of

your pharmacist.

Admission to medical institution and intravenous fluid alternative, in excessive times.

Antibiotics, if micro organism are the reason.

Pills to kill the parasites, if parasites are the reason.

Preserving off anti-vomiting or anti-diarrhoea tablets until prescribed or advocated via your medical doctor, due to the truth the ones medicinal drugs will preserve the contamination inner your body.

Danger elements

Gastroenteritis takes area everywhere in the international and may have an effect on humans of every age.

Those who can be more vulnerable to gastroenteritis include:

Younger children. Kids in infant care centers or widespread faculties can be mainly prone as it takes time for a kid's immune gadget to mature.

Older adults. Man or woman immune structures generally generally tend to end up a good deal much less green later in existence. Older adults in nursing houses are inclined due to the truth their immune systems weaken. Additionally they stay in near touch with others who can also skip along germs.

Schoolchildren or dormitory citizens.

Anywhere that agencies of humans come together in near quarters can be an surroundings for an intestinal contamination to get handed.

All people with a weakened immune tool. In case your resistance to contamination is low — for instance, if your immune machine is compromised through manner of HIV/AIDS, chemotherapy or each different clinical situation — you will be particularly at risk.

Every gastrointestinal virus has a season while it's far most lively. If you stay in the Northern Hemisphere, for example, you are much more likely to have rotavirus or norovirus infections within the winter and spring.

The precept worry of viral gastroenteritis is dehydration — a extreme lack of water and critical salts and minerals. If you're healthful and drink enough to replace fluids you lose from vomiting and diarrhea, dehydration ought to now not be a hassle.

Infants, older adults and those with weakened immune systems may additionally additionally turn out to be significantly dehydrated when they lose extra fluids than they might update. Hospitalization is probably desired just so out of place fluids can be replaced thru an IV of their fingers. Dehydration can not often bring about demise.

The pleasant way to prevent the unfold of intestinal infections is to comply with those precautions:

Get your infant vaccinated. A vaccine against gastroenteritis as a result of the rotavirus is to be had in some international locations, consisting of america. Given to kids inside the first year of existence, the vaccine appears to be effective in stopping excessive signs and symptoms of this contamination.

Wash your hands very well. And ensure your children do, too. If your children are older, educate them to easy their fingers, specifically after the use of the bathroom.

Wash your fingers after converting diapers

and in advance than getting prepared or eating food, too. It is excellent to apply warmth water and cleansing cleaning soap and to rub arms nicely for at the least 20 seconds. Wash spherical cuticles, beneath fingernails and inside the creases of the arms. Then rinse thoroughly. Carry sanitizing wipes and hand sanitizer for times whilst cleaning soap and water are not to be had.

Use separate personal objects spherical your house. Avoid sharing consuming utensils, ingesting glasses and plates. Use separate towels in the relaxation room.

Prepare meals properly. Wash all of your culmination and vegetables earlier than consuming them. Clean kitchen surfaces before making prepared meals on them. Avoid getting ready meals if you're ill.

Keep your distance. Keep away from near contact with everyone who has the virus, if possible.

Disinfect difficult surfaces. If someone in your private home has viral gastroenteritis, disinfect tough surfaces, collectively with counters, taps and doorknobs, with a aggregate of five-25 tablespoons (73 to 369 milliliters) of family bleach to one gallon (three.Eight liters) of water.

Keep away from touching laundry which can had been exposed to an epidemic. If a person in your home has viral gastroenteritis, wear gloves at the same time as touching laundry. Wash garb and bedding in hot water and dry them at the maximum up to date setting. Wash your fingers properly after touching laundry.

Check out your infant care middle. Make sure the middle has separate rooms for changing diapers and making prepared or serving meals. The room with the diaper-converting desk need to have a sink similarly to a sanitary manner to remove diapers.

Take precautions even as travelling

While you are touring in distinctive international locations, you could turn out to be unwell from inflamed food or water. You will be capable of reduce your danger via following those suggestions:

Drink best properly-sealed bottled or

carbonated water.

Avoid ice cubes because of the truth they may be crafted from inflamed water.

Use bottled water to brush your tooth.

Avoid raw meals — along with peeled quit result, raw veggies and salads — that has been touched with the resource of human hands.

Keep away from undercooked meat and fish.

CONCLUSION

Nearly everybody gets stomach flu at some point. Given that many one in all a kind viruses can reason it, you can get it more than as quickly as. Youngsters in daycare facilities and colleges and people in care centers are greater at risk of getting it from their communities, and they'll enjoy more immoderate signs and symptoms and signs and symptoms with it.

For the general public, stomach flu is unsightly however short. However for some, it can be volatile. If you contend with a infant or older man or woman with stomach flu, watch for symptoms of dehydration and live in touch with a healthcare company. Take steps to protect your self from the virus and to save you it from spreading to others.

THE END

www.ingramcontent.com/pod-product-compliance
Lightning Source LLC
Chambersburg PA
CBHW060824260726
48660CB00003B/1083